Understanding Men

How to Attract and Seduce a Man, Keep Him Interested and Turn Him On

Stephenie Roberts

© **Copyright 2019 by Stephenie Roberts - All rights reserved.**

This document is geared towards providing exact and reliable information in regards to the topic and issue covered. The publication is sold with the idea that the publisher is not required to render accounting, officially permitted, or otherwise, qualified services. If advice is necessary, legal or professional, a practiced individual in the profession should be ordered.

- From a Declaration of Principles which was accepted and approved equally by a Committee of the American Bar Association and a Committee of Publishers and Associations.

In no way is it legal to reproduce, duplicate, or transmit any part of this document in either electronic means or in printed format. Recording of this publication is strictly prohibited and any storage of this document is not allowed unless with written permission from the publisher. All rights reserved.

The information provided herein is stated to be truthful and consistent, in that any liability, in terms of inattention or otherwise, by any usage or abuse of any policies, processes, or directions contained within is the solitary and utter responsibility of the recipient reader. Under no circumstances will any legal responsibility or blame be held against the publisher for any reparation, damages, or monetary loss due to the information herein, either directly or indirectly.

Respective authors own all copyrights not held by the publisher.

The information herein is offered for informational purposes solely, and is universal as so. The presentation of the information is without contract or any type of guarantee assurance.

The trademarks that are used are without any consent, and the publication of the trademark is without permission or backing by the trademark owner. All trademarks and brands within this book are for clarifying purposes only and are the owned by the owners themselves, not affiliated with this document.

Table of Contents

Introduction

I want to thank you and congratulate you for grabbing "Understanding Men".

This book contains proven steps and strategies on how to attract a man, how to seduce him and keep him interested.

As they say *"Men are from mars, women are from Venus"* they are from different emotional planets, therefore understanding the other sex becomes difficult at times especially when you're in a relationship.

But don't worry my lovelies, here in this guide, I'll teach you each and every trick and tip to keep your men interested in you. Men always want those women, who keep on wandering in their minds all the time, whether you're starting your relationship or just seeing a guy or a housewife who wants to keep her husband interested in her, this guidebook will help you. Not only it'll help to stabilize your relationship, but also tell you different ways to keep him coming back.

See what you're doing wrong in your relationship and make things better by improving yourself and understanding the nature of men.

I hope that you'll love this book!

Chapter 1 – Know Your Worth

Know your Worth

Universally men have almost the same requirements when they look for women, or the women they idolize. Keeping the psyche of men in your mind, you can do wonders. As they say "Act like a lady and think like a man" so I suggest you to *understand* men. Men are not that hard to understand and when you'll learn and understand your guy, you'll be able to keep his attention.

They say, to see the better results change yourself. But I'd say, do not change yourself but improve yourself. Remember you can always, always improve yourself. Be a better woman, be a classy lady and not a trashy one.

Make him chase you and don't chase him

Guys never like those girls who chase them. So don't do that. Don't run after guys because if he wants to be with you, he'll make efforts by himself to be with you. Let's agree upon it, most of us have been there. Weren't we? But it's time we should stop. Girls, know this fact that you'll lose his interest if you'll chase him. Chasing is a man's duty so let him do it. Those who run after men end up losing their self-integrity and eventually become his doormat. Men place high value on things they have to work for, so let him work for you. It doesn't mean that I want you to play games with him, but let him take the charge and be a man while you're being a classy woman and let him work hard for you.

You're worth it, you're beautiful

Don't compare yourself with other women out there. Be yourself and the right guy will come and love you. If you'll love yourself, then he'll definitely love you too. Love your bad habits and good ones both.

Trust me, when you'll start being yourself you'll earn and keep his attention. For men love those girls who love being what they are. They don't want some girl who doesn't have any personality and just a reflection of somebody else. When you're going on a date, try saying these lines in front of a mirror: "You are beautiful and you deserve beautiful things" and these lines will have a very positive impact on you and you will be more confident.

What unique traits or features you have? For example if you have a pair of perfect long legs, then try to show them to him too by wearing a perfect dress.

Your unique-ness

Let's face it; there are so many beautiful women out there, isn't it? Then what will make him think that "no, I cannot leave my woman?". Your unique qualities will make him stay.

To earn a man forever or for a really long time, you have to show him what you have and other women don't. Show off your unique qualities to him. Prove him that you're worth it. So sit down for a while and think what makes you different from other women? Is it something he'll love? Think about it and you'll find the answer.

Be a determined, goal-oriented woman

Those women who don't have any goals and ambitions in life are never liked by men. Let him know that you have set many targets and you are determined to achieve those targets. In this way, you'll earn his respect. Be a lady that influences people.

Determine what you want and what you don't

If it is the starting of your relationship, then set your rules. Determine what you want from a relationship and what you don't. Remember, an amazing personality will attract an amazing guy. Determine your dos and don'ts and set your priorities.

Self confidence

Self-confidence is the key. Develop your self-confidence by telling yourself that what you have is enough. Stop thinking that your eyes are not that big and your smile makes you ugly. Tell yourself that you have so many things to be grateful for. Men always want to be with the happy girls because happy people have this capability to make the most of everything and they don't create dramas. So don't be a drama queen. Be a happy person. When you're going on a date with him, practice a little in front of a mirror how you'll start your conversation. This tip will boost your level of confidence.

Control your mood swings

Don't throw random mood swings at him; it is a big turn off. A lady knows how to control her mood swings and she doesn't let her mood to control her. If you are one of those whiny girls who cry a lot all the times, you won't be liked by him and someone else will catch his attention. So don't let anyone grab your man's attention. Try to be funny and lighten his mood by telling some jokes. I bet he'll love it.

I am not saying not to act sad in front of him, show what you feel, be expressive but don't be one of those girls who always talk about their problems in front of their men. Men slowly start losing interest in that type of women.

Done working on yourself? Alright, you are all set to seduce him with your oh-so-hot looks, in the second chapter we will tell you about how to seduce him and get his maximum attention!

Chapter 2 – How To Seduce Him

How to look beautiful to have his attention

Feeling beautiful from the inside after reading the first chapter? Well, I guess it's time for the outside part. It is very important of course to feel good and perfect from the outside too because men are more visual. They love seeing beautiful things so how to look beautiful from the outside too to be a complete package to him? Let's explore this thing here

Choosing the right dress to wear

Choose the things that look best on you because if you know how to carry your dress, you'll win his attention and he'll be impressed. Men love those women who know what to wear and how to wear it. So choose the right dress according to your height, for example if you're short then you should consider wearing those tops that are short and not very long. Short top will help you look good and you won't look short.

Show off your skinny body with a not-so-tight dress and by 'not-so-tight' I mean your dress should be tight enough to show your curves or body but not that tight to show everything you have inside. Keep him guessing and show a little. Don't wear skimpy clothes because this way he'll have wrong perceptions about you. Be careful about the color you choose to wear, because colors also play a very important part in determining mood and personality of a person. Dress up nicely and according to occasion. There's a saying *"When in doubt, wear red"*.

Wearing red is the best idea on a date. Red appeals men the most, so add a little red to what you wear. Red lipstick is a great idea and it goes with almost every color. According to a research, men find women in red more attractive than other colors, so provide some red for his eyes.

Hair

Take extra care about your hairstyle, because men love hair and it's one of the things that they notice at first date. Make the best hairstyle possible. Men love long hair because they can't have them. So if you have long hair, they will be noticed and loved by your man.

Eye contact

Eyes say a lot, and you'll be amazed to hear what eyes can do. They can make a guy fall in love with you in no time. Say it with the eyes but don't overplay it. Stare him and gaze him for a while and then look away. In this way, he'll get more curious and also you'll get his attention. Eye contact can tell you what he is currently thinking about you or whether is into you or not. Tell him your thoughts through eyes.

Lips

Lips are important when it's about turning a man on and your chances will increase if you have sexy, juicy lips. If you don't have them, don't worry it's okay. You can make them look perfect by applying hot shades of lipsticks. Get his attention by applying bright colored lipstick or you can also lick or bite them when he's looking. The more he will look at your lips, the more he'll be desperate to kiss you.

Use your smile as your weapon

Smile and laugh are the biggest weapons a woman can have. Picture two girls in your mind, one is smiling and the other one is sad. Who would you want to talk to, the smiling one, right? Yes, men would do the same. When you're talking to him, smile often. He'll think of you as a happy woman and he'll be more attracted towards you. Remember! Men don't like when you start complaining about the stuff in front of him, this gives him a wrong impression. Also, don't smile too much, just smile to seduce, not to tell him you like him. Try to be fun. Tell some jokes and laugh. Make him fall in love with your laughter.

Perfumes

According to a survey, 89% men said that the scent of women enhances their attractiveness. So, you know what this means? It means you have to be careful about selecting your perfume too. Perfume influences your judgment about the other sex subconsciously. It is one of the important factors for the success of seduction.

Also, pay special attention to all the parts of your body. Look good and smell good. Take a bath before meeting him and take proper care of your skin and body. Guys love women who love staying healthy and fit.

Femininity

If you think that a guy doesn't like femininity, you're wrong. According to males, a girl should act like a girl. This trait cannot be resisted by any masculine men. So ladies, never be shy of what you are. Embrace your femininity and show it off. They say you should act like a lady and think like a man. So ladies, make it your motto for life.

Chapter 3 – The Way To Unbelievable Sex

Flirting is healthy

Now that you have gone through the physical and inner traits to earn a man now it's time to show him what you can do sexually to him, keep on reading to find out!

How to Flirt

A little flirting is safe and healthy and a little bit of it won't harm you both. Don't be the uptight type of girl, just flirt with him like a classy lady. Smile, blush, and take his compliments with an open heart.

Play with your hair a little while talking to him and be expressive, run your fingers on his chest and flirt a little with him. Touch him to tell him that you want him and give him hints.

Flirt even when you are a married couple now. Wait for him when he arrives and when he reaches home, flirt with him. Kiss him passionately and tell him that you still love him.

A little touch game

Touch him a little for example while having dinner or some conversation. Place your fingers over his palm or let your feet touch his feet when you are sitting next to each other and pretend like you don't know what's happening. Give him opportunity to touch you a little by asking him to pass on something to you, this will arouse him sexually and he'll crave for more touch. Single touch can make a difference, ladies! So go for it!

Squeeze his hands or slap his arms while telling a joke, tell him by your gestures that you don't mind being touched by him.

If you want to grab his attention forever, never tell him that you like him too much or love him too much. Love is a dirty game, ladies! And you should know how to play it. If you let a guy know you like him without his putting any efforts, he won't be excited to have you. And whatever you'll do for him, he'll assume that you're trying so hard to get his attention and he'll feel not-so-attracted towards you. So avoid that. Always make it look like that HE's the one who's chasing you and not you, when actually it's you behind the scene.

Dance with him

Girls, you have got the body, so why not show him by a little dancing trick? So, take him to the dance floor with you, show your hot body while dancing, let him touch you, show your curves and he'll be yours. Dancing is a great way to construct sexual chemistry between you.

Whisper your thoughts

Do you feel like your man is turned off? Maybe is he losing interest in you?

I was like you before, and then I learned how to ALWAYS turn him on whenever I wanted. That's the secret:

Talk dirty to him.

Whisper your naughty thoughts to him, it'll automatically arouse him and he'll wait eagerly to get laid.

That's a great resource that helped me a lot with my boyfriend. Our sexual life was really becoming frustrating. I felt like I couldn't arouse him anymore and every day I thought I could have lost him.

Play the sexting game when you're not together. Men always love a little naughty digital flirting. Even if you're his wife, send him a sexy message when he's at work. Try texts like: "Having naughty thoughts" or send him your hot photo, but by hot I mean in sexy clothing and stuff and not naked.

Be creative for your man and he will be yours forever.

Wear sexy undergarments

Wear sexy stuff underneath, for example choose your panties and bras in the color he loves. It'll arouse him sexually at once. Ask him to buy you the fantasy item he wants you to wear.

Try to know his fantasies and create an environment he loves. Change your dressing habits a bit, if you wear jeans everyday then try to wear skirt and heels one day and surprise him with a new makeover and a hairstyle.

Love network expert Kerner says, take risks and change your approach of who you think you are and how well you do in bed. Sharing your thoughts and fantasies to him will stimulate your mind in a new way and leads to unbelievable sex.

Take it slow and set a mood before having sex. Give him a massage first, like rub his belly or anything that relaxes him. According to the author of *How Sex Works*, stress is one of the major problems that don't let men to be aroused, so he suggested all the women out there to try to minimize his stress level to have connective sex.

Try to arouse his feelings first and remind him of the love you both had at the beginning of the relationship by looking at old photos together. Kerner says it's a good trick to keep his attention and evokes a feeling of tenderness and affection.

Chapter 4 – How to Keep Him Interested

How to keep a relationship working

To have your man's attention always towards you, you'll have to work on every aspect starting from yourself and what you can give him and now it's time I tell you how to keep your man's attention. There are many things to consider keeping your man fully attracted towards you because if he wants to have only sex with you, he can have it with so many other girls, so to keep him coming you have to give him emotional stability and love too. So here are my tips!

Be the best among his social circle

Men are competitive species and they always want to be with the best woman so try to impress his friends, make them think you're the best and you've a shot.

Families

Families are very important for men and they are a little more traditional than women are so be nice with them and win everyone's heart and when they will adore you he'll start adoring you even more.

Don't hate his hobbies

Men hate when you ask them to pause Fifa, so don't. Learn to respect his hobbies and try to play with him too. He'll think that you're the complete package and won't leave you ever.

Know that you guys cannot be exactly like each other so don't hate things he loves. Remember: if he doesn't hate when you take long time to get ready and spend so much money on shopping, then you should return some favor and let him do whatever he likes doing. Let him watch football, basketball or cricket in peace and try to watch it with him too.

Pay attention to what he says

Ask him about his dreams and goals and stare him when he tells you about them, this gesture will show him that you're paying attention to him. Men loves when a girl listens to them and they love being loved as we girls do. So they'll be automatically more drawn towards the girl that listens and appreciates his man.

His space is important

Men love to have their personal space. They don't like those who are a control freak. So don't act like one. Try to understand the fact that he'll love you even more if you give him space to think and be free. If you'll show him that you respect his personal space then he'll be more attracted towards you.

Women who show men that they need them the most and sound desperate to them, men are never drawn towards them. So when you want to attract him, don't tell him that your happiness lies in his hands. Try to show him that you enjoy your life and although he is important, he's not the only happy part of your life.

Give yourself time

When you feel like things are going fine, take a step back and stop giving too much of your time to him. Take this time off and give yourself time. Men are weird; they take things very easy when it's going smooth with every girl. So in the beginning of your relationship, don't show him you're impressed by him. This will make him think more and more about you and he'll try hard to make an impression on you.

Compliment him

Just as we girls love when a man compliments us, men love it too and it boosts up their confidence and makes them happy. You should complement his accomplishments and this thing will positively affect his life and mood and he'll stay faithful to you. Don't make him feel small by comparing him with someone else and don't cry if he doesn't have much money or something. Just prove your worth by staying by his side always and I promise you he won't go anywhere.

Food

The stomach of a man is the way to his heart. Men love food and if you're a good cook, he'll definitely love you. It doesn't matter if you don't cook regularly, but cook once in a week his favorite dish and it'll make his day. It'd be better if you cook meal for the dinner because he'll be very happy to eat that hot cooked dinner that you'll cook for him after a long tiring day at work.

Make him reliant on you

A relationship works perfectly when both partners rely on each other for their needs and they last longer if both partners can give more than just sex to each other. Both partners should fulfill each other's needs so provide your guy reasons to stay with you. Give him your love, your sincerity, be there when he needs you and don't throw him out in hard times. Be the type of girl he likes because in this way he'll think that you're his dream girl or something.

Make him feel loved

Men need affection more than girls. Girls are emotionally strong species while men are not. So treat your men like he deserves to be treated. All they need from their woman is love and her attention. Make your man feel special and care about him. Love him and show him that you love him. For example when he leaves for work, give him kisses and hug him so tightly. Tell him to come back home soon and ask him to take care of himself.

A shoulder

Ask him to share problems with you. Be his shoulder and listen to his problems. It is not necessary if you provide solutions for his problems. Listening to him would be enough sometimes. Ask him about his dreams and goals and show him the way and support him to achieve things. Earn his heart and he will treat you as a goddess.

Quality time

Spend great time with your man. A time free of distractions will be loved by your man and it'll release his tension too. For example, plan some activity other than watching TV together and the usual routine. Take him to the cinema or have a dinner together.

Gifts

Everyone love gifts and so does men. It is not necessary to buy an expensive gift but a small gift can do wonders. Give him his favorite chocolate or when he is working, bring a cup of coffee for him.

Make him smile

When he is sad or depressed don't share your problems with him, it'll make him more angry and sad. Men seek peace and the women who provide that peace to them; they are attracted towards them the most.

Never talk about your past or exes

Men don't like it when women talk about their exes. They are extremely possessive by nature about their girlfriend they don't want to hear what she's been doing with all other men in the past. So, don't try to jealous him with your past stories. Learn to let the past go and love what's in front of you.

Don't be his mom

Ladies, don't act like his mother all the time. Remember he already has a mom and he doesn't need another one. So don't scold him, don't shout on him, and don't tell him what to do unless he asks you. Instead, be his best friend and his lover.

Stay faithful

Most importantly, stay loyal and stay faithful to him. Don't flirt with other men and stay true to him. Don't do things that'll hurt him. Be a classy lady and know your limits. Once you've earned his trust, he won't go anywhere.

Keep a balance between your work, love and family life

Keep your life in a perfect balance. Don't overdo things. Those women who take only their work as their priority are always at loss. Men need their time too so when he asks you to give him time, you should do it. The key to happiness is to live a balanced life and if you're a woman that gives time to everything, then you're a keeper.

Respect

Respect yourself and he'll respect you too. Don't ever lower your demands or standards for the guys, because your true guy will stick to you no matter what happens. Do not settle for less because you'll be loved by the person who truly deserves you.

Don't criticize him

If you're a woman who constantly criticizes your man then you're doing the relationship wrong. Men never like those women who constantly criticize their boyfriends or husbands. Criticism is good but over criticism is not and ladies, try to find a more polite way to tell him things. Harsh criticism will never make things better but it'll create more differences between you two.

Conclusion

Thank you again for reading this book!

I hope this short guide was able to help you find good steps and techniques to make your man happy. The next step is to always remember that a man will love you if you'll love yourself. So never stop loving yourself no matter what happens and try these tips too and you'll have his attention forever.

Thank you and good luck, my friend!

Stephenie Roberts

www.ingramcontent.com/pod-product-compliance
Lightning Source LLC
LaVergne TN
LVHW020101190726
843498LV00012B/1924